50 Fitness Myths:
Don't Believe All the Hype

By IFBB Pro April Cosimano
& Renee' Novelle

Cover design by April Cosimano

www.AprilCosimano.com

www.ReneeNovelle.com

MYTH: Genetics determine everything about your body

It would be so easy to blame our current state of health and fitness on genetics, something entirely predetermined and, therefore, absolutely and 100% out of our control. But alas, science has something else to say in the matter...

Yes, genetics play a large part in our lives. Our genetic makeup will determine our height, our eye color, certain diseases, our motivation, and the shape of our muscles. There are even several studies that prove some people with certain genetic makeups will be predisposed toward physical activities, or will respond better to different types of exercise. So it's easy to understand how genetics became the scapegoat for laziness.

However, genetics alone won't determine everything about your body.

If you have flawless genetics and a poor diet, you won't wake up with perfectly chiseled abs and slender thighs. Alternatively, if you're born with poor genetics, it doesn't mean you're doomed to live in a body you dislike. Even if you have the "fat gene", a genetic predisposition toward obesity, it doesn't mean that you're living with an invisible wall that stands between you and your road to success. A 2008 study published in the *Archives of Internal Medicine* showed that even people who possess the FTO gene were able to prevent unnecessary weight gain through regular physical activity. It may take a little more effort on your part, but any person can achieve their personal health and fitness goals with enough time and dedication.

MYTH: Great abs start in the gym

While that might make sense at first glance, the truth is that great abs actually start in the kitchen. Here's why: You can do crunches for hours a day, but if you're eating an unhealthy diet, all that definition will be lost under a blanket of fat.

Instead, start with your diet and analyze what you're putting into your body. Fine tune your menu to include a solid balance of lean protein, healthy fats and plenty of nutrients from fruits and vegetables. Couple this with core work at the gym and you'll begin to see results in a very short amount of time.

MYTH: Fasted cardio is vital to lose weight

Born in the bodybuilding community before making its way into the mainstream fitness population, fasted cardio has become the new go-to exercise to burn fat and drop weight quickly. While there *are* unmistakable benefits to fasted cardio when done correctly, as proven by numerous research studies, it can be very harmful when done incorrectly. So make sure you understand the process, and speak with your physician before attempting it.

That being said, fasted cardio isn't necessarily *vital* to lose weight. Weight-loss is achieved by an energy/calorie deficit. That means you simply have to burn more energy than you eat in order to lose weight – however you decide to do the burning. The truth is, there's no bad time to get your cardio in. Whether you're doing it on an empty stomach or not, the point is to get it in, get the calories burned and move on toward your goals.

MYTH: Cardio is the most effective fat burner

Cardio helps to burn unwanted fat, yes. And it can be a great way to get started on your weight-loss journey. But cardio alone is not enough to reach your goals. And it may not be the most effective method if you're looking for quick results.

A 2012 study performed at Duke University and published in the *Journal of Applied Physiology* showed that a healthy balance of cardio and resistance training is ideal for reducing fat mass and increasing lean muscle mass in adults, and showed more results than just cardio alone. An additional study published in 2009 in the *European Journal of Applied Physiology* suggests that those who performed weight training *prior* to cardio successfully burned more calories *during* their cardio than those who went straight to the treadmills. So keep your cardio, but add a few weight lifting exercises beforehand for the best and fastest results.

MYTH: Women who lift get bulky

Personal trainers nation wide have heard this rhetoric time and again, and it remains the number one fear most women express when starting on a new fitness program. Visions of chemically-altered female bodybuilders dance in their heads, though the reality is quite different – and can be easily proven with a little science and math.

For most women, regular weight lifting results in an increase in *strength*, not *size*. Your muscles become stronger, denser, and therefore look more defined when paired with a proper diet. However, the process of "bulking up" – or gaining extra muscle size – is a long and involved process that can take months, and requires a specific plan that's mostly calorie dependent.

In order to gain just one extra pound of muscle naturally, a woman would need to consume approximately 200 *extra calories a day* according to the Academy of Nutrition and Dietetics, and her protein intake would have to be nearly twice the recommended allowance of 46 grams made by the Institute of Medicine. Additionally, she'd have to train in a way that's specifically formulated to build muscle, which is vastly different from the common workouts that most women perform – even with a trainer.

So while it's possible for a woman to gain muscle mass during the process of working out, it's not probable if a woman is watching her diet and exercising with weights normally. The most you'd have to worry about is a well-trimmed mid-section and enviable glutes.

MYTH: You don't have to lift weights to look "fit"

We love cardio. It's a generalized way to help burn calories, increase metabolism and improve heart health among its many beneficial side effects. And there's nothing quite like banishing your workday stress with a good, long run.

But cardio alone won't give you those beautifully tight triceps or that perfectly perky derriere you're looking for, which is one of the many reasons why the Mayo Clinic recommends resistance training as part of a well-rounded exercise program. Whether you prefer lifting weights at the gym, enjoying a Pilates class while utilizing resistance bands, or using your own body weight in a boot camp class, you have to make each muscle class work in order to see an improvement in quality.

MYTH: Carbs make you fat

Sure, bad carbs will make you fat. Too many carbs in general will make you fat. But then again, too much of any food group will add on the pounds if not eaten in the correct quantities to maintain a healthy weight. Yet this is a marketing trend used all the time to sell you on the latest diet craze or food product.

The fact is, good carbs are necessary in order to maintain a properly functioning body, and you should be incorporating the correct amount of carbs into your daily diet. Studies that have been published in the *Archives of Internal Medicine* have proven that carbs are responsible for improving your mood, your brain power and your heart health, while researchers at Brigham Young University found that carbs even promote weight-loss due to the dietary fiber found in many complex carbohydrates.

So it isn't about eliminating carbs from your diet completely, but learning which carbs are healthy and which aren't. The Harvard School of Public Health suggests swapping highly processed items like white bread, fries and cookies for minimally processed whole grains, nutrient rich vegetables like broccoli, and beans. Simple, small dietary changes like this can lead to significant results down the road.

MYTH: Vegans/Vegetarians can't be bodybuilders

The number one concern voiced when discussing a plant based diet and bodybuilding always comes back to the amount of lean protein necessary to achieve the results most bodybuilders desire. While many Americans associate protein with animal-based products, it certainly isn't an exclusive source and there are many plant-based protein options to help fill in the gaps.

For example, while there are 38g of protein in 5 ounces of chicken, you can get the same amount of protein in only 6g of dried nuts, 9.5 tablespoons of natural peanut butter, 2.5 cups of tempeh, or 8 tablespoons of hempseed. Or you can supplement your food with additional plant based protein powders. So do a little research and be creative, the possibilities are endless!

MYTH: You can't drink alcohol if you want to be healthy

Alcohol is full of empty calories, and a routine nightcap could undo all that hard work you just put in at the gym. Not to mention how a morning hangover can be detrimental to your daily health routine. But that doesn't mean you necessarily have to give up alcohol completely.

If you enjoy the occasional social beverage, Boynton Health Services at the University of Minnesota recommends that you wait 4-6 hours after a workout before drinking. And be sure to replenish your body with plenty of water, food and vitamins before indulging in order to combat the effects that alcohol may have on your body – like dehydration and protein depletion.

Also, be sure to limit your intake to only 1-2 servings, and select variations that are lower on the calorie scale like a vodka soda, which has only 96 calories compared to a sugary margarita that serves up 170-680 calories depending on the size and recipe!

MYTH: Don't eat at night

Despite the long-standing Adele Davis quote, "eat breakfast like a king, lunch like a prince and dinner like a pauper", recent research studies have shown that the problem with eating at night isn't necessarily the time of day that you consume your food. Calories are calories, and as long as you're burning less than you consume, you should still be able to maintain your weight-loss goals.

The real problem with eating at night is that it's so easy to overdo portion sizes on after dinner snacks. West Virginia University reminds us that usually these snacks consist of high-calorie, fatty foods like chips, buttery popcorn or cookies. It's easy to lose track of how much you've consumed while you're socializing with friends, watching television with family or zoning out as you unwind with a book. Before you know it, you've consumed nearly an entire bag which can lead to indigestion or sleep interruption – not to mention all the unnecessary calories that add up.

Instead, plan your meals to allow for a little 100 calorie snack in the late evening if this is a habit that's important to you. And keep healthy items like a small yogurt or piece of fruit within easy reach.

MYTH: You have to take a lot of supplements to get good results

Yes, professional athletes and bodybuilders rely on a specialized diet that includes different supplements to help them take their performance to the next level. But the types and amounts of supplements they take aren't necessary for the average fitness enthusiast.

While it's true that you need more protein to increase muscle mass, the average person can get what they need to achieve their goals out of a well balanced diet that's full of lean proteins, vegetables and healthy carbs. Adding a multivitamin into your daily routine could prove beneficial to cover any lacking nutrients, but it's not necessary to include a dozen additional supplements, protein shakes or vitamins. Anyone who advertises differently is trying to sell you a product that you don't necessarily need.

MYTH: Slow metabolism keeps me fat

In truth, only a very small percentage of people have naturally high or naturally low metabolisms, according to research studies noted by the Mayo Clinic. And often this is a result of a hyperactive or draggy thyroid, both of which can be regulated with the right medications.

Research studies have shown that people who are overweight actually burn more calories than slim individuals in their day-to-day activities because bigger bodies require more calories to move around, thus they're the ones with the higher metabolism. The common problem is that people who are overweight significantly underestimate the amount of calories they've taken in for the day - sometimes by as much as 50 percent! - which leads them to consume way more than they need, states a 2004 study published in the *American Journal of Clinical Nutrition*. If you aren't counteracting that with a fair amount of physical exercise, the result is weight gain, regardless of how fast your natural metabolism is.

MYTH: Fill-in-the-blank exercise is bad for you

There are plenty of articles circulating the web that list various exercises with the claim that they are bad for you. But if you read closely enough, the problem isn't usually with the exercise itself, it's more often about the fact that average gym-goers aren't incorporating proper form when performing the exercise. This inevitably leads to injury and pain.

But any exercise has the potential to be problematic if you're using improper form. So it's vital that when you first begin your fitness journey, you enlist the help of a professional who can monitor your movements and correct bad form before it becomes a permanent habit. Also, make sure that your level of fitness is appropriate for the exercise you're attempting – some exercises are more effective and less problematic once you reach a more advanced stage. So be patient with yourself until you get there, we all have to start somewhere.

MYTH: You're drinking plenty of water

Everyone's heard the advice to drink eight glasses of water a day. And enthusiastic health devotees do their best to stick to this one-size-fits-all formula.

But recent research suggests a more individualized approach is better, and the Harvard Health Letter published new recommendations in 2015 that suggest four to six glasses of liquid are sufficient for the average person – though people who are extremely active, or are pregnant or breast feeding may need to increase that number significantly. And don't forget that liquid based foods like soup, watermelon and lettuce count toward that daily goal as well.

The Institute of Medicine, however, recommends that instead of restricting yourself to any one formula, individuals should get in tune with their bodies, monitor their body's thirst request and drink enough fluids that urine is colorless or light yellow – regardless of how may cups necessitates that result.

MYTH: Extreme weight-loss diet plans are sustainable

We love all the commercials and glossy advertisements promoting the extreme weight-loss plan *du jour* – "Lose 30 pounds in just 30 days!", "Drop 10 pounds in the first week!", "I lost 75 pounds using this method!" If there's any amount of calorie deficient built into the plan, then sure, it will work for you.

But here's the reality check – to get extreme results like that, you have to go to extreme measures. Maybe you lost 50 pounds in a month by eating only cabbage and drinking only cranberry juice, but has your diet taught you how to maintain your new weight once the program ends? Can you really see yourself sticking to this eating pattern for the rest of your life? Often times, these plans do more long-term damage than offer short-term benefits, and participants derail themselves once cravings become too strong.

Instead of embarking on a crash diet that will only serve you short-term results with no long-term plan toward sustainability, seek out the advice of a professional who can help you develop the eating habits necessary to keep the weight off for good. Remember, being healthy and achieving a body composition that reflects your healthy choices should be a lifestyle – it's not a sprint with a permanent finish line.

MYTH: Weight-loss/Fitness gains are purely physical – never a mental attitude

Yes, you have to have a balanced diet and commit to some sort of physical activity to get the most out of your efforts. These are both very physical activities that are required to make significant advancements on your health journey.

But your mental attitude and focus is just as important to your workouts as your muscles are. In a 2014 study published in the *Journal of Neurophysiology*, researchers immobilized the wrist/hands of two different groups for four weeks (similar to wearing a cast for four weeks). One group was guided through a series of mental images of strong muscle contractions five days a week, while the other group did nothing.

At the end of the study, they found the group who had performed the mental exercises retained 50% more muscle and strength than their counterparts, leading them to believe that mental imagery plays a significant role in physical development.

Apply this to your personal journey by picturing your muscles working while you use them both in the gym and outside of it. Imagine the body you've always wanted, then make strides to work toward it. This sort of mental imagery will get you half of the way toward your goals, while your physical efforts will make up the remaining balance. And your mindset will push you through even the most difficult of times if you really focus and trust yourself.

MYTH: Workouts don't need to be structured or varied

Yes, regular exercise is good for you. And maybe you've found a fitness routine that's helped you reach significant goals. But that doesn't mean you need to keep to the same workout every day for the rest of your life.

In fact, research has shown there are significant benefits to mixing things up once in a while. In addition to the mental stimulation of trying something new, adding variety to your daily routine has proven to develop new muscles, prevent injuries and break through fitness plateaus that seem to be holding you back. And by taking a little time to plan a structured workout before you hit the gym, you can ensure that you're hitting all the right parts of the body in an even manner, so you can achieve the symmetry and balanced definition you desire.

MYTH: Fat-free anything is better for you

While fat-free diet foods have been a trend since the 1990's, that doesn't mean it's the smart choice. Our bodies require a certain amount of fat to support a healthy system and appearance. Fat benefits our skin, nails, hair and boosts brain power. So restricting your diet of any and all fats is a costly mistake.

Additionally, many fat-free foods are full of chemicals like artificial sweeteners, and tend to be higher in carbs than their more natural counterparts. Instead, opt for a low-fat version if it's available, which according to the FDA and USDA must contain a healthy 3 grams of fat or less and isn't filled with the same chemical sweetening agents. Or, indulge in the full-fat option, just limit your portion so you can stay within healthy guidelines and still maintain your fitness goals.

MYTH: Stretching is useless

While recent studies performed at Florida State University and Auburn University Montgomery have been circulating that claim static stretching isn't ideal before a workout, that doesn't mean stretching should be completely thrown out of your daily routine. Just be mindful that you're doing the correct type of stretching before and after your workout to get the most from the exercise.

Dynamic stretching (stretching while the body is in motion) like arms circles and straight leg swings, are the perfect way to warm the body up before starting a difficult workout. And static stretching for five to ten minutes after your workout is the ideal way to cool your body down.

MYTH: I'm too busy/tired to workout

This is the number one excuse made by couch potatoes across the nation. And sure, it seems reasonable at first glance. You're busy with your career, working 8, 10, maybe even 12 hour days. Then there's your personal errands, family obligations, commute time and emergencies to take into account. And of course, everyone deserves a little down time or fun once in a while. Before you know it, you've completely filled your day without a minute to spare. So how could you possibly fit in an hour or so for the gym?

There's good news. You don't have to spend your entire evening inside a gym to get the results you need. In fact, you don't even have to do your workout all at once for it to be effective.

Instead, break up your routine into small, easy portions and spread them out throughout the day or week. Try to tackle 20-30 minutes of cardio first thing in the morning before you get ready for work. This will give you an extra energy boost to tackle your day, and will help you achieve all those items on your calendar. At lunch, set aside 15 minutes to do a few lunges and squats outside or in the bathroom. When you get home, spend another 15 minutes on bicep curls and shoulder lifts while dinner is in the oven. Without putting too much effort into it or sacrificing your schedule, you've just put in an hour workout that day.

Analyze your daily routine to see where you might be able to fit in a few more exercises to really give your body the boost it deserves.

MYTH: I can eat anything I want because I workout

It's a common misconception that getting 30 minutes of exercise in will magically erase all the negative side effects of your bad eating habits. And unfortunately, this is the number one reason why most people don't see any results for their hard work, despite hours spent in the gym each week.

The bottom line is that if you want to see results, you have to follow a healthy, balanced diet. Weight-loss and maintenance will always be about "calories in versus calories out", though it's easy to underestimate the number of calories you're putting into your body, and overestimate the number you're burning if you don't keep to a plan.

For example, if you run two 10 minute miles on a treadmill, you've burned just a little over 200 calories – or the equivalent of one Grande Caramel Macchiato at Starbucks, or one slice of regular cheese pizza.

Instead of indulging every day, do your best to eat clean throughout the week, and leave yourself one day on the weekend that you can enjoy some of the foods you love in moderation.

MYTH: Barely eating is a great shortcut

Many people assume that by skipping meals – and thereby saving a significant number of calories – they're tricking the system in their favor and will achieve their fitness goals faster. But this couldn't be further from the truth, and may actually work against you – especially if the meal you're skipping is breakfast.

Research has shown that people who skip meals or severely restrict their food consumption battle cravings for foods high in fat and sugar. This is because your body believes it's starving, so it will naturally crave foods that add more calories per volume to give you the energy you need to get through the day. This puts your body at risk for extreme metabolic changes that includes weight gain and an increase in glucose.

Studies have shown that those who eat smaller meals more frequently have greater success at maintaining a healthy weight and progressing toward their goals.

MYTH: There's a magic diet pill that will work

While we'd all love for this to be true, there's simply no magic pill that will allow you to eat whatever you want and shed off all your unwanted weight. Truthfully, most diet pills aren't regulated, let alone tested for safety. And many come with claims that haven't been researched or proven scientifically, though many people fall for their claims anyway.

Those who have reported a significant loss while taking the pills have generally coupled the medication with a healthier diet and moderate exercise routine. But this alone would result in weight-loss without the pill. Save yourself the money, and put in a little work to get the exact same results.

MYTH: All protein powders are created equal

Protein powder is an excellent way to pack in more nutrients without all the extra calories – especially for those pursuing a bodybuilding competition with a need to stay lean. And with a plethora of flavors, brands and varieties, it's easy to find something that you like.

But that doesn't mean that all protein powders work in the same way, or with the same benefits. To ensure you're getting exactly what you need, spend some time studying labels and ingredients, and do a little research online. For example, whey concentrates are usually packed with unnecessary fillers and tend to be a more generalized form of protein, while whey isolates are cleaner, faster absorbing and work better with low carb diets. There are a variety of options for vegans/vegetarians as well, with plant based options that speak to their specific dietary needs. Whatever your situation, make sure you have a clear understanding of what you're putting into your body, and what your body will get in return.

MYTH: Eating healthy is expensive

We've heard the "Whole Paycheck" joke when it comes to eating organic and healthy, and while there may be some truth to it, it doesn't have to be that way! Now more than ever, shoppers of healthy, organic produce have plenty of options when choosing brands they love – and with those options comes a variety in price points.

Publix, Whole Foods and others have created their own name brand products as a way to reduce costs for conscientious shoppers, and green markets - where produce is available from local farms - continue to grow in popularity. With a little research and the right strategy, purchasing healthy, organic food for your family shouldn't put a burden on your budget.

MYTH: I need a gym membership to get in shape

Here's a secret that gyms and fitness studios don't want you to know – you don't need them to get in shape.

Yes, having a membership with dozens of machines is helpful, not to mention the social aspect can be enticing. But if your budget restricts you from spending $20 a month, or you aren't comfortable yet walking into a crowd of fitness enthusiasts, all is not lost. Utilize what you have at your disposal instead, and you can give yourself just as good of a workout at home, in the park or at the beach.

Neighborhood sidewalks are great replacements to treadmills. Squats, lunges, pushups and a variety of other exercises can be done in your living room. Climb a staircase or stadium seats regularly for extra lift. Swim laps in your community pool for added cardio. A playground often has pull-up bars and other equipment that the creative individual can utilize. Whatever you choose to do, think outside the box, and don't limit yourself to what's considered a traditional workout.

MYTH: If you eat clean, you're getting enough vitamins naturally

If you're focusing on the bigger picture of your diet and eating a variety of foods from every category, this might be true. But can you really say that you're consuming enough nutrient rich foods in enough categories every day to keep up with your daily needs?

In 2010, the updated Dietary Guidelines for Americans noted 10 nutrients that most Americans may be missing, including potassium, calcium, vitamin D and vitamin C. To supplement this, make sure you're taking a quality multivitamin every day that will provide what your menu might be missing.

MYTH: Sleep has nothing to do with fitness

The theory goes something like this: when you're sleeping, you aren't actually exerting energy, performing exercise or in any other way doing something to visibly burn calories. So what does sleep have to do with fitness and maintaining a healthy weight?

Everything!

Researchers at Brigham Young University found that getting less than 6.5 hours of sleep or more than 8.5 hours of sleep was linked to higher body fat, as was poor sleep quality. Furthermore, a smaller study published in the journal *Obesity* in 2012 revealed that overweight women who were actively pursuing a weight-loss program had a 33% higher success rate when they were getting adequate, quality sleep each night.

Why? When we aren't getting enough sleep, we're drinking more caffeine (often lattes filled with sugar and fat), we're too tired to cook healthy meals and rely on fast food, we experience more cravings because our hormones are affected, we skip the gym or don't give our time there our full effort, and we lose focus on our goals. Additionally, a study from Columbia University found that when sleep-deprived, our activity is increased in the insular cortex, which regulates pleasure-seeking natures. Unhealthy food and alcohol – both packed with calories and fat – satisfy this region more than healthy choices.

MYTH: There's nothing I can do to control cravings

Yes, cravings hit suddenly and they hit hard. It can seem like they're taking control of our day if we let them. But the good news is you don't have to. By implementing a variety of techniques such as eating with others, distracting your thoughts, giving into small portions, and supplementing craved food with healthier options, you can conquer your cravings and stick to your health schedule.

But perhaps more important is understanding what your cravings actually mean. Often time, our body will tell us exactly what it needs, we just have to be mindful to interpret the clues. It could be that we need to get more sleep (fatty food cravings) or that we're experiencing high amounts of stress (salty food cravings). Or it could mean that our body is lacking a vitamin that we need.

For instance, craving sweets could mean a problem with blood sugar fluctuations. To counter this, fill your diet with more high-fiber foods to keep your blood sugar levels stable. Chocolate cravings mean you're deficient in magnesium, while a craving for red meat indicates an iron deficiency. A cheese or pizza craving indicates a fatty acid deficiency, and caffeine cravings could mean dehydration. Having a clear understanding of what our cravings *actually* mean makes it easier to combat them without giving in to temptations that could derail our progress.

MYTH: Cheat meals offer no value when trying to lose weight

Many people think that to reach their goals, they can never have those delicious foods they love again. But completely denying your body some of those foods is actually counterproductive.

Planning a single "cheat meal" or "refeed" meal that satisfies cravings while providing a balance of protein and healthy carbohydrates helps to 1.) break through weight-loss plateaus by providing a boost of calories, 2.) curbs instances of binge eating, and 3.) regulates dopamine and leptin levels. Not to mention that a cheat meal is great motivation to make sure you're getting your daily workouts in.

But this doesn't mean that you should eat anything and everything during that time. Try restricting your indulgence to a single meal, one day a week. You should also steer clear of fried foods like chicken wings and fries that could increase your cholesterol, as well as sodium drenched pizzas. Opt instead of a juicy bison burger on a whole wheat bun, or chicken fajitas with a side of black beans and rice. Or you could even try a whole wheat pasta with grilled salmon and light marinara sauce topped with plenty of vegetables.

MYTH: The amount you sweat determines the amount of calories you've burned

You've seen that person at the gym – the one wearing three layers of gym clothes beneath plastic sauna suits, climbing on the cardio equipment to try to sweat off as much fat as possible.

It's great in theory, but that's not exactly how it works. If it did, we could all sit in a sauna all day and melt our way to the ideal weight.

The National Academy of Sports Medicine reminds us that sweat isn't an indicator of how many calories you're burning, but is instead produced as a way to cool our bodies down and regulate core temperature. And since different people are born with a different number of sweat glands, and drink different quantities of water throughout the day, you could be burning hundreds of calories and never break a sweat – or you could glisten while walking through the parking lot to your car. What little bit of weight you are losing is likely from water retention and not necessarily a long term gain. Focus instead on time spent exercising and the quality of your movements for an effective session, instead of the puddle you leave behind on the gym floor.

MYTH: More gym time is better

While multiple gym sessions a day seems to be a trend among top athletes and bodybuilders, it's very possible that overdoing your workout could be counterproductive. A study from the University of Copenhagen found that those who exercised for only 30 minutes a day lost approximately 40% more weight than their counterparts who worked out for an hour or more.

Why?

Overtraining can take a toll, both mentally and physically. After just 60 minutes of exercise, ligaments, joins and muscles tend to get weak, which increases your risk of injury. And people who train for extensive amounts of time tend to be less active and more sedentary outside the gym, according to a study presented by the American College of Sports, likely from being too tired. While it's important to exercise long enough for optimal results, it's also important that you listen to your body and don't overstress it.

MYTH: Bikram yoga burns more calories than regular yoga

Bikram, or "hot" yoga, has become legendary due to the claims of thousands of calories burned in a single 90-minute session. But despite the 105-degree temperature and 40% humidity in the room, the reality may be far different from the expectation.

A study conducted at Colorado State University proved that each 90-minute session only really burns between 330-460 calories – or the equivalent to walking briskly at about 3.5 miles an hour for the same duration. And a study performed at the University of Wisconsin in 2013 found no difference in the benefits between Bikram and regular yoga since metabolic rates have been found to remain the same.

Any amount of extra calories burned and fat lost from engaging in Bikram yoga is likely a result of the 26 intense poses that participants are guided through, as well as the dedication of its fans. Any type of exercise that's done with consistency will usher better results, and Bikram yoga fans are eager to return to the studio with regularity.

MYTH: Crunches burn belly fat

Despite what late night infomercials would have you believe, performing hundreds of crunches or ab exercises will *not* burn belly fat.

What these exercises do is strengthen your core muscles and give them a nice, "toned" appearance. But crunches don't burn a significant amount of calories, nor can you spot burn fat on your body through any means. To get chiseled abs, continue to do your core exercises, but also be sure to integrate a clean diet that will reduce the layer of fat covering your muscles.

MYTH: Swimming is great for weight-loss

Swimming is great for strengthening muscles, building endurance and increasing lung capacity. And doing any type of cardio exercise is better than doing none at all. But the actual, measurable weight-loss benefits associated with swimming are inconsistent.

On one hand, we have a study published in the *American Journal of Sports Medicine* that shows subjects who followed their swimming program actually *gained* five pounds, where test subjects performing other types of cardio programs lost weight. But on the other hand, we have a study performed at the University of Utah that shows swimming is just as effective for weight-loss as many land-based exercises.

The difference seems to be in the temperature of the water, as well as the duration and difficulty of the exercise.

A study conducted in 2011 and published in *Medicine and Science in Sports and Exercise* revealed that an immersion in cold water stimulates the appetite, and as a result, these individuals eat large meals that replace all the calories they lost, negating any benefits they gained. A University of Florida study confirmed this finding, and found that while men burned the same amount of calories in cold and warm water, those who had exercised in cold water consumed 44% more calories that day than their warm water counterparts.

The buoyancy of the water, as well as swimming pace, also negates some of the effect.

If you're going to use this technique as your primary cardio for weight-loss, be sure to monitor your diet carefully, and put in enough time and effort at the pool to make the exercise effective.

MYTH: CrossFit is all you need

CrossFit is a great, full body workout when done with proper technique that will reduce the risk of injuries. But it's not a one-size-fits-all plan, and depending on your goals, you may need to incorporate other exercise techniques as well.

CrossFit focuses on building strength and endurance, which is great for the average gym goer. But if you're trying to lose a significant amount of weight, train for a marathon, work toward a bodybuilding competition or have other targeted goals, this alone will not get you where you want to go. Evaluate your goals carefully, and then put a plan in place that addresses every aspect of that goal instead of following the masses with the hope that it will work.

MYTH: You're guaranteed proper form when using machines

From the thousands of hilarious gym videos circulating YouTube demonstrating incorrect form, it's safe to say not everyone knows what they're doing in the gym – even while using the machines.

While machines don't necessarily guarantee perfect form, they are easier to learn on for people first starting out in a gym environment. And they provide a simple approach to planning your workout that doesn't require a lot of research. Though you can still get injured on a machine from incorrect form, there's often a significantly reduced risk of injury here when compared to free weight or body weight exercises.

It's still advisable to enlist the help of a professional trainer to orient yourself with proper form while using machines. Many gyms will offer a few complimentary sessions, or you can ask someone at the front to watch your form on the first round to be sure you're being safe and effective.

MYTH: No pain, no gain

Sure, everyone wants to feel a little sore after their workout. You want some reassurance that what you're doing is working, and that it's working the right muscles. But soreness itself isn't an exclusive indicator of how hard you're going in the gym, and often it can be an indicator of a bigger problem or possible injury.

Ideally, a healthy amount of muscle soreness should arrive and then begin to dissipate again within three days, and you should be able to perform the same workout again without much discomfort. If you're past the three-day mark and feel a significant amount of pain in your muscles, experience swollen limbs, feel pain in your joints, or have very dark urine, you should make an appointment with your doctor immediately.

MYTH: You can target your fat burn

Every infomercial and diet pill would love for you to believe that targeted fat loss or "spot reduction" is possible, but science begs to differ.

A study led by the University of Connecticut in 2007 tested the theory by putting over 100 participants through a 12-week resistance-training program that only exercised their dominant arm. If the "spot reduction" theory held up, they would've seen fat loss only on this limb and no where else on the body. Instead, MRI assessments of the participants revealed that fat loss was generalized throughout the body, instead of only appearing in that one area.

A similar study was repeated in 2013 and published in the *Journal of Strength & Conditioning Research*, this time putting participants through a 12-week program of leg presses using their non-dominant leg. At the end of the study, researchers again found that while the amount of overall body fat decreased, it was not localized to the one-and-only area they had been exercising.

MYTH: Don't workout on an empty stomach

This has been a highly debated subject for a long time now. On one hand, you want to eat so you don't feel fatigued during your workout. But on the other hand, it's not always possible to consume and digest a meal prior to working out. And having a stomach full of food can make some people feel nauseous during a heavy workout. Especially first thing in the morning.

While most professionals recommend eating something light 1-2 hours before hitting the weights, some studies have shown there's merit in doing cardio in the morning prior to breakfast.

Truthfully, this all depends on you. Whether you chose to eat or not should depend on how your body feels. Pay attention to the signs if your body is telling you it needs more fuel, and keep a banana or some whole grain peanut butter crackers in your gym bag just in case. But if your stomach feels better without anything in it, go for it!

Just make sure you stay well hydrated throughout your workout either way.

MYTH: You shouldn't workout every day

While rest days are vital to building muscle, and overtraining has been proven to cause injuries, this is not an excuse to skip workouts 3-4 times a week. And the type of "resting" you do depends entirely on the type of athlete you are.

Historically, our ancestors spent much of their days walking, hunting, gathering and performing other physical activities to stay alive and well. And their bodies were designed to handle this. While our schedules and culture has changed significantly over the centuries, no longer necessitating that we chase our food, our genetic makeup has stayed the same. As a general rule, our bodies need far more exercise than the average American adult gets since approximately 60% of American adults are irregular in their activities and 20% are completely sedentary, meaning they get no exercise at all other than walking between their car and office, or the couch and refrigerator.

If your workouts are already of the gentler variety – think walking, yoga, swimming – there's no real need to rest completely with a day off. These programs are designed to be gentle on joints and muscles, so there's less wear-and-tear on your body than if you were weight lifting every day.

Iron enthusiasts and bodybuilders, however, may want to step back from the weights once a week if doing a full body workout each day. Or change up your workouts so that you're alternating which body parts you're focusing on. Our bodies need approximately 48 hours to recover from an intense workout, so keep this in mind when planning in advance. That being said, it's perfectly fine to engage in some light cardio or stretching on your off days to keep your body active. Especially if you want to enjoy a little something extra during your cheat meal.

MYTH: Running beats walking

It's easy to understand why people believe this – you're moving faster while running, therefore you must be burning more calories. And yes, you are - by about twice the amount.

However, weight loss alone shouldn't be your only goal when it comes to cardio. And recent studies published in the *Journal of the American College of Cardiology* suggest that people who run most days of the week at a 7 mile an hour pace or faster actually presented the same mortality risk as sedentary people. The study went on to suggest that moving at a slower pace – a brisk walk or slower jog – would lower your death risk by 25%. This is due to the strain that long-term, intense endurance training puts on your lungs, heart, joints and immune system. The American Heart Association goes on to report that moderately paced walking is just as effective when it comes to reducing blood pressure, cholesterol levels, diabetes risks and heart disease. Researches from the Lawrence Berkeley National Laboratory in California investigated the National Runners' Health Study and discovered that those who had accomplished the same distances – regardless of how long it took them to get there – gained comparable health benefits to each other.

So do what feels right to you, and challenge yourself when you're ready. But move forward with the understanding that if you're looking at the bigger picture of your health journey, you don't have to succumb to the "only-running-works" lifestyle.

MYTH: Protein bars/drinks are great meal supplements

This depends on the bar you choose, and you're going to have to look closely at the nutrition labels to make sure you're selecting the right one.

The fact is, most protein bars might as well be a Snickers, and most protein drinks could pass for a Starbucks latte when it comes to calories and sugar provided. Many smaller bars have over 400 calories and more than 30 grams of sugar, with little nutritional value to offset that. That's way more than any person needs to consume for a meal, not to mention you're missing out on all the vitamins and minerals your body gets from "real" food.

If you're going to treat them as a meal supplement, start by thoroughly analyzing the ingredients so you can make sure you're getting as many benefits as possible while eliminating unnecessary ingredients. And limit your supplementing activity so this is more the exception than the rule in your health life.

MYTH: All calcium comes from dairy

We've been drilled since childhood to believe that to get the amount of calcium we need for strong bones and muscles, we have to drink milk. And lots of it. To get the recommended 1,000mg a day, that's three 8oz glasses!

But the reality is there are plenty of non-dairy foods filled with calcium. Collard greens provide 268mg per 1 cup of cooked leaves, and broccoli rabe provides 100mgs in a 2/3 cup serving. One cup of raw kale gives you 101mgs, and ½ cup of dried figs offers 121mgs. Some fish, like sardines and salmon, are even high in calcium, boasting 351mgs and 463mgs respectively in one can! Vegans and vegetarians may already know that tofu is both a source of protein *and* a source of calcium, giving consumers 434mgs per half cup.

Just doing a little research and adding more variety to your normal menu can offer you all the calcium you need without turning to dairy based products.

MYTH: Fruit can't make you fat

We wish!

Fruit is great – it provides an amazing source of vitamins, it offers high amounts of natural fiber, and it contains natural sugars to keep blood sugar levels stable...when eaten correctly.

However, fruit is still high in calories, carbohydrates and fructose - especially if you're noshing on dried fruit, which packs five to eight times more calories and sugar than the fresh variety! So fruit isn't exactly a "free" food like many think. It's easy to derail your diet with just one apple and one banana a day – which would pack in 57 grams of carbohydrates, or more than half of your daily carb allotment.

Like all foods, enjoy your fruit. Just eat it in moderation, and opt for fresh whenever possible.

MYTH: I'm too old to get fit

Only 25% of people between the ages of 65-74 are exercising regularly, partly due to the myth that they're too old to start a fitness regime. But they're wrong.

Alicia Arbaje, MD, MPH at the Johns Hopkins University School of Medicine reminds us that many of the symptoms that we associate with old age, like weakness and loss of balance, are actually just signs of inactivity. And these have nothing to do with the process of aging itself.

In fact, because exercising even at a moderate level promotes strength, balance and agility, and boosts memory power that prevents dementia, older individuals are *encouraged* to implement some form of exercise into their daily routines. Individuals who have heeded the call can be found running marathons well into their 70's, stepping onto the bodybuilding competition stage in their 80's, and boat rowing in their 90's.

These aren't fitness freaks of nature; these are individuals determined not to allow their age to define them. Will you?

MYTH: Gluten-free foods are better for everyone

The most recent food craze would have you believing that gluten is poison for everyone. And yes, if you have celiac disease or gluten sensitivity, gluten can cause a major health concern. But that doesn't mean that everyone should avoid grains all together.

According to Celiac Central, only about 1% of the population suffers from true celiac disease – a condition that affects the regenerative capacity of the intestines. When those diagnosed with this disease consume gluten, it can cause damage to the intestines. And since the organs can't repair themselves as easily as others, they tend to suffer through some painful side effects. Those with gluten sensitivity make up another 6% of the population, and are affected by similar intestinal symptoms, just without the physical damage.

That being said, more than 93% of the population has absolutely no adverse reactions to gluten at all. Those who have self-diagnosed themselves as a way to jump on the new trend are actually robbing themselves of the natural vitamins and minerals that whole grain products (usually made from wheat, rye or barley) supply.

Cutting back on carbs as a dietary measure is one thing, but eating gluten-free foods all the time just isn't necessary without a medical diagnosis.

MYTH: It's all about the scale

We're all guilty of it. We set a certain goal for our weight loss or health, and check the scale regularly to track our progress. We're hoping for a significant drop in numbers, and if we don't get it, we'll make serious adjustments in our formula – or give up all together.

But what most people forget is that a pound of fat weighs the same as a pound of muscle. Most people are exercising while dieting, which means they're building muscle while losing fat. So naturally, the scale won't move too much until you've reached the end of your goal.

Instead of focusing so much on the scale, focus instead of the size of your clothes and the way your body feels. If you feel tighter all around and your clothes are fitting more loosely, then consider it a successful week and don't put so much pressure on yourself to make that scale move.

MYTH: Juicing is a great way to get a shot of nutrients

Yes, juicing is a great way to get a healthy dose of nutrients into your system quickly, especially if you aren't too keen on eating large quantities of fruits and vegetables.

However, when you juice you lose much of the fiber and nutrients that you could get from eating the fruit whole. That's because most of these nutrients are found in the pulp and skin of fruits and vegetables. And this is discarded in the juicing process.

You also have to be mindful of the amount of calories you're putting into your drink. As noted previously, fruit tends to be high in sugar and calories. Juicing just 4 to 5 cups of fruit (the average amount for one serving of juice) packs in up to 600 calories a serving, so adding too much in a concentrated potion could have reverse effects. Instead, use mainly vegetables for your base concoction, then throw in a single apple or orange for a little flavor.

MYTH: Thin on the outside, healthy on the inside

You may not workout or eat particularly healthy, but you do well enough that you still look good in a bathing suit, and your BMI is within the normal range. So you must be healthy, right?

Wrong!

The term "skinny fat" is starting to gain momentum outside the gym as well as inside. And this is a very dangerous place to be in the health world.

To break it down, an individual may appear to be slim and in good shape. They don't have any obvious rolls around their belly, and they could easily fit into a size of clothing that the average American would envy. So they think they get a pass on healthy eating and exercise. This is where they get into trouble.

On closer inspection, they're actually metabolically obese. And according to a study published in the *Journal of the American Medical Association*, approximately one-in-four thin people suffer from pre-diabetes as a result of this. Those who progress to become fully diagnosed with diabetes have twice the risk of death as their overweight, diabetic counterparts.

Weight alone isn't an indicator of high blood pressure or insulin levels. And the insulin, the fat storage hormone, is where the damage stems from. Leaving this unchecked could not only lead to diabetes, but also heart attack, stroke, dementia and even cancer. We highly recommend that even thin individuals visit their doctors regularly for a check-up. And make sure proper blood testing is done to monitor insulin and lipid levels. Stay on track with a healthy, balanced diet, and get some sort of movement into your exercise plan for at least 30 minutes every day.

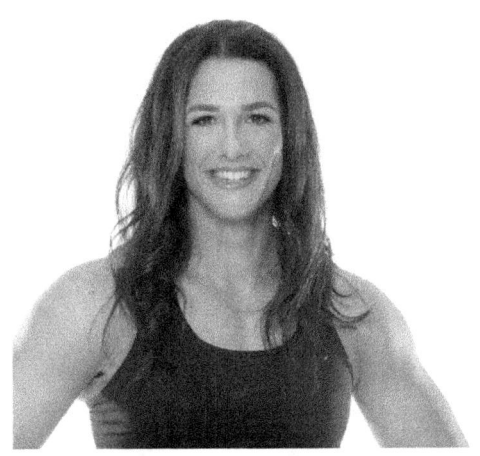

About IFBB Pro April Cosimano

April Cosimano has provided her training skills to facilities such as Gold's Gym, LA Fitness in Bonita Springs, FL and Fort Myers, FL among others. Throughout her influential career, she has been fortunate enough to train in Muay Thai Kickboxing with Crafton Wallace- UFC fighter, as well as several notable men and women bodybuilders.

In 2014, April earned her IFBB Pro status in Women's Physique at the esteemed NPC National Bodybuilding Championships in Miami, Florida. This was following her performance at the NPC Southern States Championship in July 2014 where she placed 1st in Women's Physique Master's, 1st in Women's Physique Open, and took 1st place Overall for Women's Physique. In her first show, the 2013 NPC South Florida Competition, she also placed 1st in Women's Physique Tall and 1st in Women's Physique Overall. In 2015, she took her passion a step further and co-founded the online health, fitness & bodybuilding magazine, beLegendary Magazine.

By incorporating all of these experiences into her programs, she has provided well rounded, effective methods of training. She has had the pleasure of including Abercrombie & Fitch models, Miami Dolphins cheerleaders, Hollywood celebrities, individuals prepping for fitness and bodybuilding competitions, individuals prepping for the FBI Physical Fitness Test, and Police Academy applicants amongst her clients, as well as scores of other men and women on the journey of accomplishing their personal health goals. April has helped them ALL transform their bodies into the best they can be.

www.AprilCosimano.com

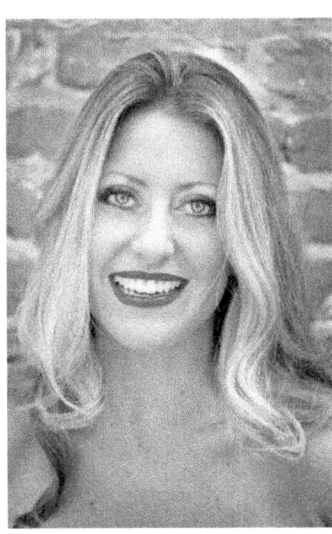

About Renee' Novelle

Following in her family's footsteps, Renee' Novelle cultivated a passion for writing at a very young age. While some of her early works earned local awards and recognition, it wasn't until well after college - where she earned a full dance scholarship at age 15 - that she followed her interest with fervor.

Beginning in 2008, Novelle pursued journalism and has found placement for hundreds of articles in both print and online publications. Additionally, she has written multiple screenplays, has contributed her effective writing style to many non-profit and for profit organizations, and has 10 books to her credit.

In 2015, she partnered with IFBB Pro April Cosimano to develop beLegendary Magazine, which focuses on health, fitness and bodybuilding competition advice, as well as true-life inspirational stories.

Though she received her Bachelor's of Science in Communication, *summa cum laude*, she considers herself a constant student of the written word. She's an avid reader, an enthusiastic quote poster, and rarely takes "no" as a final answer. She believes in following dreams, and that in the end, you always end up where you're meant to be.

www.ReneeNovelle.com